Table Of Contents

Chapter 1: Understanding Depression and Anxiety

The Link Between Nutrition and Mental Health

In recent years, there has been a growing recognition of the powerful link between nutrition and mental health. Research has shown that the food we eat can have a direct impact on our mood, energy levels, and overall mental well-being. In this subchapter, we will explore the connection between nutrition and mental health, and how making mindful food choices can help manage depression and anxiety.

One of the key ways in which nutrition can influence mental health is through the production of neurotransmitters, the chemical messengers that regulate mood and emotions in the brain. Certain nutrients, such as omega-3 fatty acids, B vitamins, and amino acids, are essential for the synthesis of these neurotransmitters. By including these nutrients in our diet, we can support the production of feel-good chemicals like serotonin and dopamine, which can help alleviate symptoms of depression and anxiety.

Additionally, a diet rich in whole, nutrient-dense foods can provide the body with the energy and nutrients it needs to function optimally. When we eat a diet high in processed foods, sugar, and unhealthy fats, we may experience fluctuations in blood sugar levels and inflammation, which can contribute to mood swings and feelings of anxiety. By focusing on whole foods like fruits, vegetables, whole grains, and lean proteins, we can stabilize our energy levels and support our mental health.

Moreover, nutrition plays a crucial role in gut health, which has been increasingly linked to mental health. The gut-brain axis is a bidirectional communication system between the gut and the brain, and research has shown that imbalances in gut bacteria can contribute to mood disorders like depression and anxiety. By consuming probiotic-rich foods like yogurt, kefir, and fermented vegetables, as well as prebiotic foods like bananas, onions, and garlic, we can support a healthy gut microbiome and promote mental well-being.

In conclusion, the link between nutrition and mental health is undeniable. By making mindful food choices and prioritizing a diet rich in nutrients, we can support our mental health and well-being. Whether you are a parent, teenager, adult, student, nutritionist, life coach, personal trainer, public speaker, blogger, content maker, influencer, or simply a regular person, incorporating these principles into your diet can help you manage depression and anxiety more effectively. Additionally, restaurant owners and resort owners can play a significant role in promoting mental health by offering nutritious, balanced options on their menus. Let's work together to prioritize our mental health through mindful eating and nutrition.

Common Symptoms of Depression and Anxiety

In this subchapter, we will explore the common symptoms of depression and anxiety that many individuals may experience. It is important to recognize these symptoms in order to seek proper treatment and support for mental health challenges. By understanding the signs of depression and anxiety, individuals can take proactive steps towards managing their mental well-being.

One common symptom of depression is persistent feelings of sadness or hopelessness. People experiencing depression may have a general sense of emptiness or despair that impacts their daily life. They may also lose interest in activities they once enjoyed and struggle to find pleasure in things that used to bring them joy. Additionally, individuals with depression may have changes in appetite, sleep patterns, and energy levels.

Anxiety is characterized by excessive worry or fear that is difficult to control. People with anxiety may experience racing thoughts, restlessness, and physical symptoms such as sweating, trembling, or rapid heartbeat. They may also have difficulty concentrating or feel irritable and on edge. It is common for individuals with anxiety to avoid certain situations or activities that trigger their anxious feelings.

Other common symptoms of depression and anxiety include difficulty in making decisions, changes in weight, irritability, and physical symptoms such as headaches or stomach issues. It is important to note that these symptoms can vary from person to person and may manifest differently in each individual. Seeking professional help from a therapist, counselor, or mental health provider is crucial in addressing these symptoms and developing a personalized treatment plan.

For individuals struggling with depression and anxiety, incorporating mindfulness-based practices, exercise, and a balanced diet can be beneficial in managing symptoms and improving overall mental well-being. Mindful eating, in particular, can help individuals become more aware of their relationship with food and how it impacts their mood and energy levels. By practicing mindfulness during meals, individuals can cultivate a greater sense of self-awareness and make healthier food choices that support their mental health.

In conclusion, recognizing and understanding the common symptoms of depression and anxiety is essential for individuals seeking to manage their mental health challenges. By being mindful of these symptoms and seeking appropriate support, individuals can take positive steps towards improving their well-being and living a more fulfilling life. Through mindfulness-based practices, exercise, and proper nutrition, individuals can empower themselves to overcome depression and anxiety and cultivate a greater sense of mental wellness.

How Mindful Eating Can Impact Mental Health

Mindful eating is a practice that involves paying attention to the present moment while consuming food, without judgment or distraction. This technique can have a profound impact on mental health, particularly for those struggling with depression and anxiety. By practicing mindful eating, individuals can develop a greater awareness of their eating habits, emotions, and triggers, leading to a more positive relationship with food and a reduction in symptoms of mental illness.

For parents, teaching children and teenagers the importance of mindful eating can help instill healthy habits early on and promote a positive body image. By encouraging mindful eating practices at home, parents can help prevent disordered eating behaviors and promote a healthy relationship with food. For adults and students, practicing mindful eating can help reduce stress and anxiety levels, improve digestion, and promote overall well-being. By being more present and attentive during meals, individuals can better regulate their emotions and make healthier food choices.

Nutritionists and life coaches can incorporate mindful eating techniques into their counseling sessions to help clients better manage their depression and anxiety. By teaching clients how to tune into their hunger cues, emotions, and physical sensations while eating, nutritionists can help individuals develop a greater awareness of their eating patterns and make more mindful food choices. Personal trainers and public speakers can also promote mindful eating as a tool for mental health management, encouraging clients to practice mindfulness during meals and snacks to support their overall well-being.

For bloggers, content makers, and influencers in the niches of mindfulness-based depression anxiety management, depression anxiety management through exercise and physical activity, and nutrition and diet for depression anxiety management, discussing the benefits of mindful eating can provide valuable insight and resources for their audiences. By sharing personal experiences, tips, and strategies for incorporating mindful eating into daily routines, these individuals can help others improve their mental health and well-being. Additionally, restaurant owners and resort owners can support mindful eating practices by offering mindful eating menus, workshops, and resources for guests looking to enhance their mental health through nutrition and mindfulness.

Overall, incorporating mindful eating into daily routines can have a positive impact on mental health for individuals of all ages and backgrounds. By practicing mindfulness while eating, individuals can develop a greater awareness of their thoughts, emotions, and behaviors surrounding food, leading to improved mental health outcomes. Whether you are a parent, teenager, adult, student, nutritionist, life coach, personal trainer, public speaker, blogger, content maker, influencer, or restaurant or resort owner, incorporating mindful eating practices into your daily routine can help support your mental health and well-being.

Chapter 2: Mindfulness-Based Depression Anxiety Management

Introduction to Mindfulness Practices

Mindfulness has become a popular practice for managing stress, anxiety, and depression in today's fast-paced world. In this subchapter, we will explore the basics of mindfulness and how it can be used as a tool for improving mental health. Whether you are a parent looking for ways to help your teenager cope with anxiety, a nutritionist seeking to incorporate mindfulness into your practice, or a regular person looking for ways to reduce stress, this chapter is for you.

Mindfulness is the practice of being present in the moment and fully aware of your thoughts, feelings, and surroundings without judgment. It involves paying attention to your breath, sensations in your body, and the sounds around you. By practicing mindfulness, you can learn to quiet your mind, reduce anxiety, and improve your overall mental well-being. In this subchapter, we will introduce you to some simple mindfulness practices that you can start incorporating into your daily routine.

One of the key benefits of mindfulness is its ability to help individuals cope with depression and anxiety. Research has shown that mindfulness-based interventions can reduce symptoms of depression and anxiety by helping individuals become more aware of their negative thought patterns and emotions. By practicing mindfulness, individuals can learn to respond to stressors in a more calm and rational way, leading to improved mental health outcomes.

For those interested in incorporating mindfulness into their diet and nutrition practices, mindfulness eating can be a powerful tool for managing depression and anxiety. Mindful eating involves paying attention to the sensations of eating, such as the taste, texture, and smell of your food. By practicing mindfulness while eating, you can become more attuned to your body's hunger and fullness cues, leading to healthier eating habits and improved mental well-being.

In the following chapters, we will delve deeper into how mindfulness practices can be combined with nutrition, exercise, and other lifestyle factors to create a holistic approach to managing depression and anxiety. Whether you are a nutritionist, personal trainer, blogger, or simply someone looking for ways to improve your mental health, incorporating mindfulness practices into your daily routine can have a profound impact on your overall well-being. Stay tuned for more tips and strategies on how to incorporate mindfulness into your life for better mental health.

Mindful Eating Techniques for Managing Depression and Anxiety

In today's fast-paced and stressful world, it's not uncommon for individuals to experience feelings of depression and anxiety. These mental health issues can have a profound impact on one's ability to function on a day-to-day basis, making it essential to find effective coping mechanisms. One technique that has been gaining popularity in the mental health community is mindful eating. By practicing mindfulness while consuming food, individuals can not only improve their physical health but also manage their mental health more effectively.

Mindful eating involves paying full attention to the sensory experience of eating, including the taste, texture, and smell of the food. By focusing on the present moment and being fully aware of the act of eating, individuals can cultivate a sense of calm and reduce feelings of stress and anxiety. This technique can be particularly beneficial for those struggling with depression and anxiety, as it promotes a sense of mindfulness and self-awareness that can help individuals better understand and manage their emotions.

One of the key benefits of mindful eating for managing depression and anxiety is its ability to promote a healthy relationship with food. Many individuals who struggle with mental health issues may turn to food as a source of comfort or distraction, leading to unhealthy eating habits and potential weight gain. By practicing mindful eating, individuals can become more in tune with their body's hunger and fullness cues, making it easier to make informed and balanced food choices.

In addition to promoting a healthier relationship with food, mindful eating can also help individuals better regulate their emotions. When individuals are mindful of their eating habits, they are better able to identify triggers that may lead to emotional eating or binge eating episodes. By being present in the moment and fully aware of their emotions, individuals can develop healthier coping mechanisms for managing stress and anxiety, reducing the likelihood of turning to food as a crutch.

Overall, mindful eating can be a powerful tool for individuals looking to manage their depression and anxiety. By cultivating a sense of mindfulness and self-awareness around food, individuals can improve their relationship with food, regulate their emotions, and reduce feelings of stress and anxiety. Whether you are a parent, teenager, adult, student, nutritionist, life coach, personal trainer, public speaker, blogger, content maker, influencer, regular person, restaurant owner, or resort owner, incorporating mindful eating techniques into your daily routine can have profound benefits for your mental health and overall well-being.

Incorporating Mindfulness into Daily Life

Incorporating mindfulness into daily life can have a profound impact on our mental health and overall well-being. Mindfulness is the practice of being fully present and engaged in the moment, without judgment. By bringing mindfulness into our daily routines, we can reduce stress, anxiety, and depression, and improve our overall quality of life.

One way to incorporate mindfulness into daily life is through mindful eating. This involves paying attention to the flavors, textures, and sensations of each bite of food, as well as being aware of our hunger and fullness cues. By practicing mindful eating, we can develop a healthier relationship with food and improve our digestion and nutrient absorption.

Another way to incorporate mindfulness into daily life is through mindfulness-based exercises and physical activities. By focusing on the sensations of our body as we move, we can improve our physical fitness and reduce stress and anxiety. Mindful movement practices such as yoga, tai chi, and qigong can help us develop greater body awareness and mindfulness.

In addition to mindful eating and mindful movement, practicing mindfulness in everyday activities such as walking, driving, and even cleaning can help us cultivate a greater sense of presence and peace. By bringing our attention to the present moment, we can reduce rumination and worry, and improve our ability to cope with stress and anxiety.

Overall, incorporating mindfulness into daily life can have a transformative effect on our mental health and well-being. By practicing mindfulness in our eating, movement, and everyday activities, we can develop greater self-awareness, compassion, and resilience, and improve our overall quality of life. Whether you are a parent, teenager, adult, student, nutritionist, life coach, personal trainer, public speaker, blogger, content maker, influencer, restaurant owner, or resort owner, incorporating mindfulness into your daily routine can benefit not only your own mental health but also those around you.

Chapter 3: Nutrition and Diet for Depression Anxiety Management

Nutrient-Rich Foods for Mental Health

In this subchapter, we will explore the importance of nutrient-rich foods for mental health and how they can help in managing depression and anxiety. It is essential to understand that what we eat directly affects our mood, energy levels, and overall well-being. By incorporating a variety of nutrient-rich foods into our diet, we can support our mental health and improve our quality of life.

First and foremost, it is crucial to include foods rich in omega-3 fatty acids in our diet. Omega-3s are known for their anti-inflammatory properties and have been shown to reduce symptoms of depression and anxiety. Sources of omega-3s include fatty fish like salmon, walnuts, chia seeds, and flaxseeds. By incorporating these foods into our meals, we can support our brain health and improve our mental well-being.

In addition to omega-3s, it is important to include plenty of fruits and vegetables in our diet. These foods are rich in vitamins, minerals, and antioxidants that can help reduce inflammation in the body and support overall mental health. Berries, leafy greens, citrus fruits, and cruciferous vegetables are all excellent choices for improving mood and reducing symptoms of depression and anxiety.

Furthermore, incorporating whole grains and lean proteins into our diet can also support mental health. Whole grains like quinoa, brown rice, and oats provide a steady source of energy and can help stabilize blood sugar levels, which is essential for maintaining a balanced mood. Lean proteins like chicken, turkey, tofu, and legumes provide important amino acids that are necessary for neurotransmitter production, which can help regulate mood and reduce symptoms of depression and anxiety.

Overall, by focusing on nutrient-rich foods in our diet, we can support our mental health and improve our overall well-being. Whether you are a parent, teenager, adult, student, nutritionist, life coach, personal trainer, public speaker, blogger, content maker, influencer, regular person, restaurant owner, or resort owner, incorporating these foods into your meals can have a significant impact on managing depression and anxiety. By making mindful choices about what we eat, we can nourish our bodies and minds and live a happier, healthier life.

Meal Planning for Mood Stability

Meal planning is a crucial aspect of maintaining mood stability, especially for individuals struggling with depression and anxiety. By carefully selecting and preparing meals that nourish both the body and mind, individuals can better manage their symptoms and improve their overall mental health. In this subchapter, we will explore the importance of meal planning for mood stability and provide practical tips for incorporating mindful eating practices into daily life.

One of the key components of meal planning for mood stability is focusing on nutrient-dense foods that support brain health. Foods rich in omega-3 fatty acids, such as salmon, walnuts, and flaxseeds, have been shown to reduce inflammation in the brain and improve mood. Additionally, incorporating plenty of fruits and vegetables into meals provides essential vitamins and minerals that support overall mental well-being. By prioritizing these nutrient-dense foods in meal planning, individuals can better manage their symptoms of depression and anxiety.

In addition to choosing foods that support mental health, it is important to pay attention to meal timing and portion sizes. Eating regular, balanced meals throughout the day can help stabilize blood sugar levels and prevent mood swings. It is also important to listen to hunger and fullness cues to avoid overeating or undereating, as these behaviors can negatively impact mood stability. By practicing mindful eating and paying attention to hunger cues, individuals can better regulate their emotions and improve their overall mental health.

Meal planning for mood stability also involves incorporating a variety of flavors and textures into meals to enhance the sensory experience of eating. Including a mix of sweet, savory, crunchy, and creamy foods can stimulate the taste buds and provide a sense of satisfaction and pleasure during mealtimes. By savoring the flavors and textures of each meal, individuals can cultivate a greater appreciation for food and improve their overall mood and well-being.

In conclusion, meal planning for mood stability is a crucial aspect of managing depression and anxiety through nutrition. By focusing on nutrient-dense foods, meal timing, portion sizes, and sensory experiences, individuals can better support their mental health and improve their overall quality of life. By incorporating mindful eating practices into daily life, individuals can take control of their mental well-being and cultivate a healthier relationship with food.

How to Maintain a Balanced Diet for Optimal Mental Health

In order to maintain optimal mental health, it is crucial to prioritize a balanced diet that nourishes both the body and the mind. A diet rich in whole foods, fruits, vegetables, lean proteins, and healthy fats can help regulate mood, improve energy levels, and reduce symptoms of anxiety and depression. By making mindful food choices and incorporating a variety of nutrients into your meals, you can support your mental well-being and overall health.

One key aspect of maintaining a balanced diet for optimal mental health is to focus on whole, unprocessed foods. These foods are rich in vitamins, minerals, and antioxidants that can help combat inflammation and oxidative stress in the brain, which are linked to mood disorders like depression and anxiety. By avoiding processed foods high in sugar, unhealthy fats, and artificial ingredients, you can better regulate your mood and support your mental health.

Another important component of a balanced diet for optimal mental health is to include a variety of nutrients that support brain function and neurotransmitter production. Omega-3 fatty acids found in fatty fish, flaxseeds, and walnuts are essential for brain health and have been shown to reduce symptoms of depression and anxiety. Additionally, foods high in magnesium, zinc, and B vitamins can help regulate mood and reduce stress levels. By incorporating these nutrients into your diet, you can support your mental health and well-being.

In addition to focusing on whole foods and nutrient-dense ingredients, it is important to practice mindful eating habits that can help regulate your appetite, reduce stress, and improve digestion. By paying attention to your hunger cues, eating slowly, and savoring each bite, you can better control your food intake and make healthier choices. Mindful eating can also help you become more aware of emotional eating triggers and develop a healthier relationship with food.

Overall, maintaining a balanced diet for optimal mental health is essential for managing symptoms of depression and anxiety. By focusing on whole, nutrient-dense foods, incorporating brain-boosting nutrients, and practicing mindful eating habits, you can support your mental well-being and improve your overall health. Whether you are a parent, teenager, adult, student, nutritionist, life coach, personal trainer, public speaker, blogger, content maker, influencer, regular person, restaurant owner, or resort owner, prioritizing a balanced diet can positively impact your mental health and quality of life.

Chapter 4: Depression Anxiety Management Through Exercise and Physical Activity

The Benefits of Exercise for Mental Health

Regular physical exercise has long been known to have a positive impact on overall health, but its benefits extend far beyond just physical well-being. In fact, exercise has been shown to have a significant impact on mental health as well. In this subchapter, we will explore the various ways in which exercise can benefit mental health, particularly in the management of depression and anxiety.

One of the key benefits of exercise for mental health is its ability to boost mood and reduce symptoms of depression and anxiety. Physical activity releases endorphins, which are natural chemicals in the brain that act as mood elevators. Regular exercise can help alleviate feelings of sadness, anxiety, and stress, leading to improved mental well-being. In fact, studies have shown that individuals who engage in physical activity on a regular basis are less likely to experience symptoms of depression and anxiety.

Exercise also helps to improve cognitive function and reduce cognitive decline. Physical activity has been shown to increase blood flow to the brain, which can enhance memory, focus, and overall brain function. In addition, exercise promotes the growth of new brain cells and improves the connections between existing cells, which can help protect against cognitive decline as we age. By incorporating regular exercise into your routine, you can not only improve your mental health but also boost your cognitive function.

Furthermore, exercise can help reduce stress and improve sleep quality, both of which are important factors in managing depression and anxiety. Physical activity helps to reduce levels of the body's stress hormones, such as cortisol, and promotes the release of feel-good neurotransmitters, such as serotonin and dopamine. This can help individuals feel more relaxed and calm, leading to better sleep quality and overall mental well-being. By incorporating exercise into your daily routine, you can better manage stress and improve your ability to cope with the challenges of daily life.

In addition to these benefits, exercise can also help build self-esteem and improve self-confidence. Engaging in physical activity can help individuals set and achieve goals, which can boost feelings of accomplishment and self-worth. As individuals see improvements in their physical strength, endurance, and overall fitness, they are likely to feel more confident in their abilities to overcome challenges and achieve success in other areas of their lives. By incorporating exercise into your routine, you can improve your self-esteem and cultivate a more positive self-image.

Overall, the benefits of exercise for mental health are vast and far-reaching. By incorporating regular physical activity into your routine, you can improve your mood, cognitive function, stress levels, sleep quality, and self-esteem. Whether you are a parent looking to support your child's mental health, a student seeking to manage stress and anxiety, or a nutritionist or personal trainer working with clients to improve their well-being, exercise can be a powerful tool in promoting mental health and overall wellness. Start incorporating exercise into your daily routine today and experience the positive impact it can have on your mental health.

Types of Physical Activities for Managing Depression and Anxiety

In this subchapter, we will explore the various types of physical activities that can help in managing depression and anxiety. It is important to understand that physical activity plays a crucial role in improving mental health and well-being. By incorporating different types of physical activities into your daily routine, you can effectively combat symptoms of depression and anxiety.

One of the most popular forms of physical activity for managing depression and anxiety is aerobic exercise. This includes activities such as running, swimming, cycling, and dancing. Aerobic exercise helps to increase the production of endorphins, which are chemicals in the brain that act as natural painkillers and mood elevators. By engaging in regular aerobic exercise, you can experience a significant reduction in feelings of sadness and anxiety.

Strength training is another type of physical activity that can be beneficial for managing depression and anxiety. By lifting weights or using resistance bands, you can build muscle strength and improve your overall physical health. Strength training has been shown to increase self-esteem and confidence, which can help in reducing symptoms of depression and anxiety. Additionally, the sense of accomplishment that comes from completing a challenging strength training workout can boost your mood and improve your mental well-being.

Yoga and Pilates are two forms of physical activity that focus on mindfulness and relaxation. These practices involve gentle stretching exercises, controlled breathing, and meditation techniques. By incorporating yoga or Pilates into your routine, you can reduce stress, improve your flexibility, and enhance your mental clarity. These mind-body exercises are particularly effective in managing symptoms of depression and anxiety, as they promote relaxation and self-awareness.

Outdoor activities such as hiking, gardening, or playing sports can also be beneficial for managing depression and anxiety. Spending time in nature has been shown to reduce stress levels and improve mood. By engaging in outdoor activities, you can connect with the natural world and experience a sense of peace and tranquility. Additionally, participating in group sports or recreational activities can help you build social connections and foster a sense of community, which is important for maintaining good mental health.

In conclusion, there are many different types of physical activities that can help in managing depression and anxiety. Whether you prefer aerobic exercise, strength training, yoga, outdoor activities, or group sports, it is important to find an activity that you enjoy and can commit to on a regular basis. By incorporating physical activity into your daily routine, you can improve your mental health, reduce symptoms of depression and anxiety, and enhance your overall well-being.

Creating an Exercise Routine for Mental Wellness

Creating an exercise routine for mental wellness is essential for managing depression and anxiety. Regular physical activity has been shown to have numerous benefits for mental health, including reducing stress, improving mood, and increasing feelings of well-being. In this subchapter, we will explore the importance of exercise in managing depression and anxiety, as well as provide practical tips for creating an exercise routine that promotes mental wellness.

One of the key benefits of exercise for mental health is its ability to reduce stress and improve mood. When we engage in physical activity, our bodies release endorphins, which are chemicals that act as natural painkillers and mood elevators. This can help to alleviate symptoms of depression and anxiety, and promote a sense of well-being. Additionally, exercise can help to reduce levels of the stress hormone cortisol, which can contribute to feelings of anxiety and tension.

When creating an exercise routine for mental wellness, it is important to choose activities that you enjoy and that fit your lifestyle. This will help to ensure that you are more likely to stick with your routine and reap the benefits of regular physical activity. Some people may prefer high-intensity workouts like running or weightlifting, while others may enjoy more low-impact activities like yoga or swimming. The key is to find activities that you find enjoyable and that you can incorporate into your daily routine.

In addition to choosing activities that you enjoy, it is also important to set realistic goals for your exercise routine. This could be as simple as committing to going for a walk every day, or as ambitious as training for a marathon. By setting achievable goals, you can build confidence and motivation, and gradually increase the intensity and duration of your workouts as you progress.

Overall, creating an exercise routine for mental wellness is an important aspect of managing depression and anxiety. By engaging in regular physical activity that you enjoy, setting realistic goals, and incorporating exercise into your daily routine, you can improve your mood, reduce stress, and promote overall well-being. Whether you are a parent, teenager, adult, student, nutritionist, life coach, personal trainer, public speaker, blogger, content maker, influencer, regular person, restaurant owner, or resort owner, incorporating exercise into your routine can have a positive impact on your mental health.

Chapter 5: Implementing Mindful Eating in Daily Life

Tips for Practicing Mindful Eating at Home

In this subchapter, we will explore some practical tips for practicing mindful eating at home. Mindful eating is a powerful tool for managing depression and anxiety, as it helps us to be more present and connected to our food, our bodies, and our emotions. By incorporating mindful eating practices into your daily routine, you can develop a healthier relationship with food and improve your mental well-being.

One tip for practicing mindful eating at home is to create a calm and peaceful eating environment. Turn off the TV, put away your phone, and sit down at a table to eat without distractions. This will allow you to focus on the taste, texture, and aroma of your food, as well as your body's hunger and fullness cues. By eating mindfully in a tranquil setting, you can savor your meals and feel more satisfied, reducing the likelihood of emotional eating.

Another tip is to slow down and savor each bite. Take the time to chew your food thoroughly and pay attention to the flavors and sensations in your mouth. By eating slowly and mindfully, you can better appreciate the nourishment and pleasure that food provides, leading to a greater sense of satisfaction and contentment. This can help prevent overeating and promote a healthier relationship with food.

Additionally, it can be helpful to practice gratitude before meals. Take a moment to express gratitude for the food on your plate, the hands that prepared it, and the nourishment it provides for your body. Cultivating a sense of gratitude can enhance your eating experience and increase your awareness of the abundance in your life, reducing feelings of stress and anxiety. By approaching meals with a grateful mindset, you can transform eating into a positive and nourishing ritual.

Furthermore, listening to your body's hunger and fullness signals is essential for mindful eating. Before you eat, check in with yourself to determine how hungry you are on a scale from 1 to 10. Eat when you are moderately hungry and stop when you are comfortably full. By tuning into your body's natural cues, you can avoid overeating, honor your hunger and fullness, and maintain a balanced relationship with food. This can help you feel more in control of your eating habits and support your mental health and well-being.

In conclusion, practicing mindful eating at home can be a transformative experience for managing depression and anxiety. By creating a peaceful eating environment, savoring each bite, expressing gratitude, and listening to your body's signals, you can develop a healthier relationship with food and enhance your mental well-being. These tips can be beneficial for parents, teenagers, adults, students, nutritionists, life coaches, personal trainers, public speakers, bloggers, content makers, influencers, regular people, restaurant owners, and resorts owners interested in mindfulness-based depression anxiety management, depression anxiety management through exercise and physical activity, and nutrition and diet for depression anxiety management. By incorporating mindful eating practices into your daily routine, you can cultivate a more mindful and nourishing approach to eating that supports your mental health and overall well-being.

Mindful Eating Strategies for Dining Out

In today's fast-paced society, dining out has become a common occurrence for many individuals. While dining out can be a fun and enjoyable experience, it can also pose challenges for those who are trying to manage their mental health, particularly individuals dealing with depression and anxiety. Mindful eating strategies can be a helpful tool for navigating the dining out experience in a way that supports mental health and overall well-being.

One of the key principles of mindful eating is awareness of one's internal cues for hunger and fullness. When dining out, it can be easy to get caught up in the excitement of trying new foods or the social aspect of dining with others, leading to mindless eating. By tuning into your body's signals of hunger and fullness, you can avoid overeating and make choices that support your mental health goals.

Another important aspect of mindful eating when dining out is paying attention to the quality of your food choices. Many restaurant meals are high in processed ingredients, unhealthy fats, and added sugars, which can negatively impact mood and energy levels. By choosing whole, nutrient-dense foods when dining out, you can support your mental health and overall well-being.

Mindful eating also involves savoring and enjoying your food fully. When dining out, take the time to appreciate the flavors, textures, and aromas of your meal. Eating slowly and mindfully can help you feel more satisfied and prevent the urge to overeat. It can also enhance the dining experience and promote a sense of relaxation and enjoyment.

Lastly, practicing gratitude and mindfulness while dining out can enhance the overall experience and support mental health. Take a moment to express gratitude for the food on your plate, the people you are dining with, and the experience of trying new flavors and cuisines. By cultivating a mindset of gratitude and mindfulness, you can elevate the dining out experience and promote a sense of well-being and contentment.

How to Encourage Mindful Eating in Children and Teens

In today's fast-paced world, it can be easy for children and teens to fall into the trap of mindless eating. With distractions such as smartphones, tablets, and television, many young people are eating without paying attention to what they are putting into their bodies. This can lead to a host of negative health consequences, including obesity, poor nutrition, and mental health issues such as depression and anxiety. As parents, educators, and health professionals, it is crucial that we teach our children and teens the importance of mindful eating.

One way to encourage mindful eating in children and teens is to lead by example. As adults, we can demonstrate the importance of eating mindfully by setting aside dedicated time for meals, sitting down at a table without distractions, and savoring each bite of food. By showing our children and teens how to eat mindfully, we can help them develop healthier eating habits that will last a lifetime.

Another way to encourage mindful eating in children and teens is to involve them in the meal planning and preparation process. By including young people in decisions about what to eat, shopping for ingredients, and cooking meals together, we can help them develop a greater appreciation for the food they are eating. This hands-on approach can also help children and teens learn about the nutritional value of different foods and make better choices when it comes to their diet.

It is also important to teach children and teens about the connection between food and mood. Research has shown that certain nutrients, such as omega-3 fatty acids and antioxidants, can have a positive impact on mental health and help alleviate symptoms of depression and anxiety. By educating young people about the benefits of a healthy diet for their mental well-being, we can empower them to make better food choices and take control of their mental health.

Lastly, creating a positive and supportive eating environment is key to encouraging mindful eating in children and teens. By promoting a relaxed atmosphere during meals, avoiding negative food talk or body shaming, and encouraging open communication about food choices, we can help young people develop a healthy relationship with food. By fostering a positive eating environment, we can support children and teens in making mindful food choices that nourish their bodies and minds.

Chapter 6: Overcoming Obstacles and Challenges

Dealing with Emotional Eating Triggers

Emotional eating is a common coping mechanism for dealing with stress, anxiety, and depression. It involves using food as a way to soothe difficult emotions or distract from negative feelings. However, it can lead to unhealthy eating habits and weight gain, which can further exacerbate mental health issues. In this subchapter, we will explore strategies for identifying and managing emotional eating triggers to support better mental health outcomes.

One of the first steps in dealing with emotional eating triggers is to become more mindful of your eating habits. Pay attention to when and why you are reaching for food. Are you eating because you are actually hungry, or are you trying to avoid uncomfortable emotions? By becoming more aware of your eating patterns, you can start to identify the triggers that lead to emotional eating episodes.

Another important strategy for managing emotional eating triggers is to find alternative coping mechanisms for dealing with difficult emotions. Instead of turning to food for comfort, try engaging in activities that help you relax and unwind, such as meditation, exercise, or spending time in nature. By finding healthier ways to manage stress and anxiety, you can reduce the urge to turn to food for emotional support.

It can also be helpful to create a supportive environment that encourages healthy eating habits. This could involve stocking your kitchen with nutritious foods, planning meals ahead of time, and avoiding keeping trigger foods in the house. By setting yourself up for success, you can make it easier to resist the temptation to emotionally eat when you are feeling overwhelmed.

In addition to these strategies, seeking support from a therapist, nutritionist, or other mental health professional can be beneficial in addressing emotional eating triggers. They can help you explore the underlying issues that contribute to emotional eating and develop personalized strategies for managing your emotions in a healthier way. By addressing the root causes of emotional eating, you can make positive changes to support your mental health and overall well-being.

Overall, by becoming more mindful of your eating habits, finding alternative coping mechanisms, creating a supportive environment, and seeking professional support, you can learn to manage emotional eating triggers more effectively. This can lead to improved mental health outcomes and a greater sense of well-being. By taking proactive steps to address emotional eating, you can support your journey towards better mental health and overall wellness.

Managing Stress and Emotional Resilience

In today's fast-paced world, stress and emotional resilience have become more important than ever. Managing stress is essential for maintaining mental health and overall well-being. In this subchapter, we will discuss strategies for managing stress and building emotional resilience through mindful eating.

One of the key ways to manage stress is through mindfulness. Mindful eating involves paying attention to the present moment while eating, focusing on the taste, texture, and smell of food. This practice can help individuals become more aware of their emotions and how they are affected by food. By being mindful of what we eat, we can better regulate our emotions and reduce stress levels.

In addition to mindful eating, physical activity is another important tool for managing stress and building emotional resilience. Exercise has been shown to release endorphins, which are chemicals in the brain that act as natural painkillers and mood elevators. Regular physical activity can help reduce stress, anxiety, and depression, while also improving overall mental health.

Nutrition plays a crucial role in managing stress and emotional resilience. Eating a well-balanced diet rich in fruits, vegetables, whole grains, and lean proteins can help regulate mood and energy levels. Avoiding processed foods, sugary snacks, and excessive caffeine can also help reduce stress and anxiety. By fueling our bodies with nutritious foods, we can support our mental health and emotional well-being.

In conclusion, managing stress and building emotional resilience are essential for maintaining mental health in today's fast-paced world. By incorporating mindful eating, physical activity, and a balanced diet into our daily routines, we can better regulate our emotions and reduce stress levels. It is important for parents, teenagers, adults, students, nutritionists, life coaches, personal trainers, public speakers, bloggers, content makers, influencers, regular people, restaurant owners, and resort owners to prioritize their mental health and well-being through these strategies. Mindful eating, exercise, and nutrition are powerful tools for managing stress and promoting emotional resilience in those struggling with depression and anxiety.

Seeking Professional Help and Support

In times of struggle with mental health issues such as depression and anxiety, it is crucial to seek professional help and support. While mindfulness practices, exercise, and nutrition can all play a significant role in managing these conditions, the guidance and expertise of trained professionals can provide invaluable tools and resources to help individuals navigate their journey towards mental wellness.

Nutritionists can play a vital role in supporting individuals with depression and anxiety by creating personalized meal plans that can help balance mood-regulating neurotransmitters in the brain. By working closely with a nutritionist, individuals can learn how to incorporate foods rich in vitamins, minerals, and omega-3 fatty acids that are known to have a positive impact on mental health. Additionally, nutritionists can provide education on mindful eating practices, which can help individuals develop a healthier relationship with food and improve their overall well-being.

Life coaches and personal trainers can also offer valuable support to individuals struggling with depression and anxiety. Life coaches can provide guidance on setting and achieving goals, managing stress, and developing healthy coping mechanisms. Personal trainers can help individuals incorporate regular exercise into their routine, which has been shown to have a positive impact on mental health by releasing endorphins and reducing feelings of anxiety and depression.

For individuals looking for additional support, public speakers, bloggers, content creators, and influencers can provide valuable insight and inspiration through their platforms. By sharing personal stories, tips, and advice on managing depression and anxiety, these individuals can help others feel less alone in their struggles and provide motivation to seek help and make positive changes in their lives.

Restaurant and resort owners can also play a role in supporting individuals with depression and anxiety by offering healthy menu options and wellness programs that promote mental well-being. By creating a supportive environment that values mental health and self-care, these establishments can help individuals feel more comfortable seeking help and support in their journey towards improved mental wellness.

Chapter 7: Integrating Mindful Eating into Professional Settings

Mindful Eating Strategies for Nutritionists and Dietitians

In this subchapter, we will explore some mindful eating strategies specifically tailored for nutritionists and dietitians who are working with clients struggling with depression and anxiety. As experts in the field of nutrition, it is crucial for us to understand the impact that food and eating habits can have on mental health. By incorporating mindful eating practices into our recommendations, we can help our clients improve their overall well-being and manage their symptoms more effectively.

One important mindful eating strategy for nutritionists and dietitians to consider is helping clients develop a greater awareness of their hunger and fullness cues. Many individuals with depression and anxiety may have a disordered relationship with food, leading them to either overeat or undereat as a coping mechanism. By encouraging clients to tune into their bodies and learn to recognize when they are truly hungry or full, we can help them develop a healthier relationship with food and make more balanced choices.

Another key strategy is to encourage clients to slow down and savor their meals. In today's fast-paced world, many people rush through their meals without truly enjoying or appreciating the experience. By guiding clients to eat more mindfully, we can help them cultivate a greater sense of gratitude and pleasure in their food, which can have a positive impact on their mood and overall well-being.

Additionally, nutritionists and dietitians can help clients practice mindful eating by encouraging them to engage all of their senses during meals. This may involve encouraging clients to pay attention to the colors, textures, and flavors of their food, as well as the sounds and smells in their environment. By bringing a greater level of awareness to the eating experience, clients can enhance their enjoyment of food and become more attuned to their body's needs.

Lastly, it is important for nutritionists and dietitians to help clients cultivate a non-judgmental attitude towards food and eating. Many individuals with depression and anxiety may struggle with feelings of guilt or shame around their food choices, which can further exacerbate their symptoms. By promoting self-compassion and acceptance, we can help clients develop a healthier relationship with food and ultimately improve their mental health outcomes. By incorporating these mindful eating strategies into our practice, we can support our clients in making positive changes to their diet and lifestyle that can have a lasting impact on their mental health.

Incorporating Mindful Eating into Coaching and Training Programs

In recent years, the practice of mindful eating has gained popularity as a way to improve overall health and well-being. This practice involves paying attention to the sensory experience of eating, such as the taste, texture, and smell of food, as well as being aware of hunger and fullness cues. By incorporating mindful eating into coaching and training programs, individuals can develop a healthier relationship with food and improve their mental health.

For parents looking to instill healthy eating habits in their children, incorporating mindful eating into family meals can be a beneficial strategy. By teaching children to pay attention to their hunger and fullness cues, parents can help prevent overeating and promote a positive relationship with food. Additionally, parents can model mindful eating behaviors for their children, leading by example and reinforcing the importance of being present during meals.

Teenagers and adults who struggle with depression and anxiety can also benefit from incorporating mindful eating into their daily routines. Research has shown that mindfulness-based practices, such as mindful eating, can help reduce symptoms of depression and anxiety by promoting self-awareness and emotional regulation. By being present and focused during meals, individuals can cultivate a sense of calm and reduce stress levels, leading to improved mental health.

For students looking to improve their focus and concentration, incorporating mindful eating into their study routines can be a game-changer. By taking the time to eat mindfully, students can enhance their cognitive abilities and improve their academic performance. Additionally, by being present and attentive during meals, students can reduce their risk of emotional eating and improve their overall well-being.

Nutritionists, life coaches, personal trainers, public speakers, bloggers, content makers, influencers, regular people, restaurant owners, and resort owners can all benefit from incorporating mindful eating into their coaching and training programs. By promoting mindful eating practices, these professionals can help their clients develop a healthier relationship with food and improve their mental health. Whether through workshops, seminars, or individual coaching sessions, incorporating mindful eating into programs can lead to lasting changes in behavior and mindset. By emphasizing the importance of being present and attentive during meals, individuals can cultivate a sense of mindfulness that extends beyond the dinner table and into all aspects of their lives.

Promoting Mindful Eating in Restaurants and Resorts

In today's fast-paced world, it can be challenging to eat mindfully, especially when dining out at restaurants or resorts. However, promoting mindful eating in these settings can have a significant impact on our mental health. By being present and aware of our food choices, we can better manage symptoms of depression and anxiety.

One way to promote mindful eating in restaurants and resorts is to encourage patrons to slow down and savor each bite. This can be achieved by taking the time to appreciate the flavors, textures, and aromas of the food. By focusing on the present moment, individuals can cultivate a sense of gratitude and connection to their meals, which can help alleviate feelings of stress and overwhelm.

Another important aspect of promoting mindful eating in these settings is to provide healthy and balanced menu options. Restaurant and resort owners can work with nutritionists to develop dishes that are not only delicious but also nourishing for the body and mind. By offering a variety of nutrient-dense foods, patrons can make choices that support their mental health and overall well-being.

It is also essential for restaurant and resort staff to be educated on the benefits of mindful eating and how to support patrons in making mindful food choices. By providing training and resources for employees, establishments can create a culture of mindfulness that extends beyond the dining experience. This can help create a supportive environment for individuals seeking to manage their depression and anxiety through nutrition.

Overall, promoting mindful eating in restaurants and resorts can have a positive impact on mental health for individuals of all ages and backgrounds. By incorporating mindfulness practices into our dining experiences, we can cultivate a deeper connection to our food, our bodies, and our overall well-being. Through education, awareness, and support, we can create a more mindful approach to eating that benefits not only our mental health but our physical health as well.

Chapter 8: Sustaining Mental Wellness Through Mindful Eating

The Long-Term Benefits of Mindful Eating

In today's fast-paced world, it's easy to get caught up in the hustle and bustle of daily life and forget to take a moment to truly appreciate the food we eat. Mindful eating is a practice that encourages individuals to slow down and savor each bite, paying attention to the flavors, textures, and sensations that come with each meal. While the benefits of mindful eating may not be immediately apparent, there are numerous long-term advantages that can have a positive impact on mental health.

One of the long-term benefits of mindful eating is improved digestion. When we rush through our meals or eat on the go, we are more likely to experience indigestion, bloating, and other gastrointestinal issues. By taking the time to chew our food slowly and mindfully, we can help our bodies better break down and absorb nutrients, leading to improved digestion and overall gut health.

Additionally, mindful eating can help individuals better regulate their appetite and maintain a healthy weight. By paying attention to hunger and fullness cues, we can avoid overeating and make healthier food choices. This can be especially beneficial for individuals struggling with emotional eating or disordered eating patterns, as mindful eating can help them develop a more positive relationship with food.

Furthermore, practicing mindful eating can help reduce stress and anxiety. When we are fully present and focused on our meals, we are less likely to engage in mindless snacking or emotional eating as a way to cope with stress. By being more mindful of our eating habits, we can cultivate a greater sense of awareness and self-control, leading to reduced feelings of anxiety and a greater sense of calm.

For individuals struggling with depression, mindful eating can also have a positive impact on mood and mental well-being. By nourishing our bodies with wholesome, nutrient-dense foods and approaching meals with a sense of mindfulness and gratitude, we can help support our mental health and improve overall mood. Mindful eating can also help individuals become more attuned to the connection between diet and mental health, empowering them to make healthier choices that support their emotional well-being.

In conclusion, the long-term benefits of mindful eating extend far beyond just physical health. By incorporating mindful eating practices into our daily lives, we can improve digestion, regulate appetite, reduce stress and anxiety, and support mental well-being. Whether you are a parent, teenager, adult, student, nutritionist, life coach, personal trainer, public speaker, blogger, content maker, influencer, regular person, restaurant owner, or resort owner, incorporating mindfulness into your eating habits can help you lead a healthier, happier life.

Maintaining Mental Health with a Mindful Eating Lifestyle

In today's fast-paced world, many of us struggle to maintain a healthy balance between our mental well-being and our dietary habits. However, by adopting a mindful eating lifestyle, we can effectively manage our depression and anxiety symptoms while also nourishing our bodies with the nutrients they need to thrive. Mindful eating involves paying close attention to the sensations we experience while eating, such as the taste, texture, and smell of our food, as well as our feelings of hunger and fullness.

One of the key benefits of mindful eating for mental health is that it helps us develop a greater sense of self-awareness and control over our emotions. By tuning into our body's signals and practicing mindfulness during meals, we can better regulate our mood and reduce the likelihood of emotional eating or bingeing. This can be particularly helpful for individuals who struggle with depression and anxiety, as it can provide a sense of empowerment and agency in managing their symptoms.

In addition to promoting emotional regulation, mindful eating can also improve our overall relationship with food and our bodies. By approaching meals with a sense of curiosity and non-judgment, we can cultivate a greater appreciation for the nourishing qualities of our food and develop a more positive mindset towards eating. This can be especially beneficial for individuals who have a history of disordered eating or negative body image, as it can help them reframe their thoughts and behaviors around food in a healthier way.

For parents and teenagers, adopting a mindful eating lifestyle can be a valuable tool for promoting positive mental health and body image. By modeling mindful eating habits and encouraging open communication around food and emotions, parents can help their children develop a healthy relationship with food from a young age. Similarly, teenagers can benefit from learning how to tune into their body's signals and practice mindfulness during meals, which can help them navigate the challenges of adolescence with greater self-awareness and resilience.

Overall, incorporating mindful eating practices into our daily lives can have a profound impact on our mental health and well-being. Whether you are a nutritionist, life coach, personal trainer, public speaker, blogger, content creator, influencer, restaurant owner, or resort owner, promoting mindful eating as a tool for depression and anxiety management can help support individuals in achieving a more balanced and fulfilling lifestyle. By prioritizing self-care and nourishment through mindful eating, we can cultivate a greater sense of peace, connection, and vitality in our lives.

Inspiring Others to Prioritize Mental Wellness through Mindful Eating

In today's fast-paced world, it can be easy to overlook the importance of our mental wellness. As a nutritionist specializing in depression and anxiety management, I have seen firsthand the powerful impact that mindful eating can have on our overall well-being. By practicing mindfulness in our food choices, we can not only nourish our bodies but also support our mental health.

One of the key ways to inspire others to prioritize mental wellness through mindful eating is by leading by example. As parents, teenagers, adults, students, nutritionists, life coaches, personal trainers, public speakers, bloggers, content makers, influencers, regular people, restaurant owners, and resort owners, we can all make a conscious effort to choose whole, nutrient-dense foods that support our mental health. By sharing our own experiences and successes with mindful eating, we can inspire others to make positive changes in their own lives.

Another way to inspire others to prioritize mental wellness through mindful eating is by educating them on the connection between food and mood. Research has shown that certain nutrients, such as omega-3 fatty acids, magnesium, and vitamin D, play a crucial role in supporting mental health. By incorporating these foods into our diets and highlighting their benefits, we can empower others to make informed choices that support their mental well-being.

Additionally, by creating a supportive and encouraging environment, we can inspire others to prioritize mental wellness through mindful eating. Whether it's hosting cooking classes, sharing recipes, or simply offering a listening ear, we can help others navigate the challenges of mental health and nutrition. By fostering a sense of community and connection, we can empower others to make positive changes in their lives.

Ultimately, by prioritizing mental wellness through mindful eating, we can create a ripple effect that extends beyond ourselves. As individuals and as a collective, we have the power to inspire others to make healthier choices that support their mental health. By coming together as a community of parents, teenagers, adults, students, nutritionists, life coaches, personal trainers, public speakers, bloggers, content makers, influencers, regular people, restaurant owners, and resort owners, we can create a culture of mental wellness that benefits us all.

Chapter 9: Resources for Further Learning and Support

Recommended Books and Websites

In this subchapter, we will explore some recommended books and websites that can provide valuable information and resources for those interested in mindful eating for mental health. Whether you are a parent looking to help your child with depression and anxiety, a teenager struggling with mental health issues, or an adult seeking ways to manage your own mental health, these resources can offer guidance and support.

One highly recommended book is "The Mindful Way Through Depression" by Mark Williams, John Teasdale, Zindel Segal, and Jon Kabat-Zinn. This groundbreaking book offers practical advice and mindfulness techniques for managing depression and anxiety. It provides readers with tools to cultivate self-awareness, reduce stress, and improve overall mental well-being through mindful eating and other mindfulness practices.

Another excellent resource is the website Mindful.org, which offers a wealth of articles, videos, and guided meditations on mindfulness-based depression and anxiety management. This website is a valuable tool for anyone looking to incorporate mindfulness into their daily routine and improve their mental health through mindful eating practices.

For those interested in depression and anxiety management through exercise and physical activity, the book "The Exercise Cure" by Jordan Metzl is highly recommended. This book explores the powerful connection between physical activity and mental health, offering practical advice on how to use exercise as a tool for managing depression and anxiety.

Additionally, the website Healthline.com offers a variety of articles and resources on nutrition and diet for depression and anxiety management. From tips on incorporating mood-boosting foods into your diet to meal planning for mental health, this website provides valuable information for anyone looking to improve their mental well-being through mindful eating practices.

Overall, these recommended books and websites can serve as valuable tools for parents, teenagers, adults, students, nutritionists, life coaches, personal trainers, public speakers, bloggers, content makers, influencers, regular people, restaurant owners, and resort owners interested in mindfulness-based depression and anxiety management, depression and anxiety management through exercise and physical activity, and nutrition and diet for depression and anxiety management. By incorporating the principles of mindful eating into your daily routine, you can take positive steps towards improving your mental health and overall well-being.

Professional Organizations and Support Groups

Professional organizations and support groups play a crucial role in providing resources and assistance to individuals struggling with mental health issues such as depression and anxiety. These groups offer a sense of community and understanding that can be incredibly beneficial for those seeking help and guidance in managing their conditions. Whether you are a parent, teenager, adult, student, nutritionist, life coach, personal trainer, public speaker, blogger, content maker, influencer, or just a regular person looking for support, there are numerous organizations and groups available to assist you on your journey to improved mental health.

For those interested in mindfulness-based depression and anxiety management, organizations like the Mindfulness-Based Cognitive Therapy (MBCT) Association offer resources and support for individuals looking to incorporate mindfulness practices into their daily lives. These groups often provide workshops, retreats, and online resources to help individuals learn how to better manage their symptoms through mindfulness techniques such as meditation and body scan exercises.

If you are someone who prefers to manage depression and anxiety through exercise and physical activity, organizations like the Anxiety and Depression Association of America (ADAA) may be a good fit for you. These groups often provide information on the benefits of exercise for mental health, as well as tips and resources for incorporating physical activity into your daily routine. Whether you prefer yoga, running, weightlifting, or any other form of exercise, these organizations can help you find the right activities to support your mental health.

Nutrition and diet also play a significant role in managing depression and anxiety, and there are numerous organizations and support groups dedicated to helping individuals improve their mental health through healthy eating habits. Groups like the International Society for Nutritional Psychiatry Research (ISNPR) offer resources and information on the impact of nutrition on mental health, as well as tips and recipes for incorporating mood-boosting foods into your diet. Whether you are a nutritionist, restaurant owner, or just someone looking to make healthier food choices, these organizations can provide valuable support and guidance.

In addition to professional organizations, there are also numerous support groups available for individuals looking to connect with others who are experiencing similar struggles with depression and anxiety. Whether you prefer in-person meetings or online forums, support groups can offer a sense of community and understanding that can be incredibly valuable in your mental health journey. By connecting with others who share your experiences, you can gain insights, advice, and support that can help you better manage your symptoms and improve your overall well-being. Whether you are a parent, teenager, adult, student, or anyone else struggling with depression and anxiety, reaching out to professional organizations and support groups can be a valuable step in your journey towards improved mental health.

Continuing Education Opportunities for Mental Health and Nutrition Professionals

In today's fast-paced world, it is crucial for mental health and nutrition professionals to stay updated on the latest research and techniques in order to provide the best care for their clients. Continuing education opportunities play a vital role in ensuring that professionals are well-equipped to address the complex issues surrounding depression and anxiety management. By attending workshops, conferences, and seminars, professionals can expand their knowledge and skills, ultimately improving the quality of care they provide to their clients.

One of the key benefits of continuing education opportunities is the opportunity to learn about the latest developments in the field of mindfulness-based depression and anxiety management. Mindfulness practices have been shown to be highly effective in reducing symptoms of depression and anxiety, making them an essential tool for mental health professionals. By staying informed about the latest research and techniques in mindfulness-based therapy, professionals can better support their clients in their journey towards improved mental health.

Additionally, continuing education opportunities provide professionals with the chance to learn about the role of nutrition and diet in depression and anxiety management. Research has shown that certain nutrients and dietary patterns can have a significant impact on mental health, making nutrition an important aspect of overall wellness. By attending workshops and seminars on nutrition and diet for depression and anxiety management, professionals can gain valuable insights into how to incorporate dietary interventions into their practice to support their clients' mental health.

For parents, teenagers, adults, students, and individuals struggling with depression and anxiety, understanding the importance of nutrition and mindfulness practices in mental health management can be life-changing. By seeking out professionals who have undergone continuing education in these areas, individuals can receive the most up-to-date and effective care possible. Whether it be through individual therapy, group sessions, or online resources, professionals who have expanded their knowledge through continuing education opportunities can provide clients with the tools they need to thrive.

In conclusion, continuing education opportunities play a crucial role in ensuring that mental health and nutrition professionals are equipped to provide the best care possible for their clients. By staying informed about the latest research and techniques in mindfulness-based depression and anxiety management, as well as nutrition and diet for mental health, professionals can offer their clients the support they need to overcome their struggles with depression and anxiety. For individuals seeking help with their mental health, it is important to seek out professionals who have undergone continuing education in these areas to receive the most effective care possible.

In "Mindful Eating for Mental Health: A Nutritionist's Guide to Depression and Anxiety Management," we've explored the profound connection between what we eat and our mental well-being. Through the lens of mindfulness, we've uncovered how our relationship with food can significantly impact our mental health. By adopting mindful eating practices, individuals can cultivate a deeper awareness of their bodies, emotions, and the foods they consume, leading to improved mental clarity, emotional resilience, and overall well-being.

 Throughout this journey, we've delved into practical strategies for incorporating mindfulness into our eating habits, such as tuning into hunger and fullness cues, savoring each bite, and being mindful of the origins and impacts of our food choices. We've also examined the role of nutrition in managing depression and anxiety, highlighting the importance of a balanced diet rich in nutrients that support brain health.

 Furthermore, we've discussed the potential pitfalls of modern food environments, where processed foods laden with additives and sugars often dominate. By embracing mindful eating, individuals can navigate these challenges more effectively, making informed choices that nourish both body and mind.

As we conclude our exploration, it's evident that mindful eating is not just about what we put on our plates; it's a holistic approach to nourishing ourselves on every level. By cultivating mindfulness in our eating habits, we can foster a deeper connection with ourselves, promote mental clarity and emotional balance, and embark on a journey toward greater overall well-being.